DISCOVER THE ROOTS TO YOUR ANGER

by

Mark D. Chapman

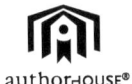
authorHOUSE®

AuthorHouse™ UK Ltd.
500 Avebury Boulevard
Central Milton Keynes, MK9 2BE
www.authorhouse.co.uk
Phone: 08001974150

© 2008 Mark Chapman. All rights reserved.

No part of this book may be reproduced, stored in a retrieval system, or transmitted by any means without the written permission of the author.

First published by AuthorHouse 10/22/2008

ISBN: 978-1-4343-8809-4 (hc)
ISBN: 978-1-4343-8808-7 (sc)

Printed in the United States of America
Bloomington, Indiana

This book is printed on acid-free paper.

DISCOVER THE ROOTS TO YOUR ANGER

A Complete Treatment Guidebook

An invaluable guide for anyone interested in improving their personal development skills.

Mark D Chapman – Chartered & Licensed Psychologist with the

The British Psychological Society & South African Health Council Profession

Picture: Cape Point South Africa

'**Discover the Roots to Your Anger**' presents a framework that includes helping you overcome unhelpful angry outbursts. Drawing on his own clinical experience, Mark Chapman, a Clinical Psychologist, suggests ways to face up to our anger in practical ways. Using skills of discussion, reflection, support and active listening, people are helped to confront their feelings and thoughts associated with their anger and frustration. A combination of ideas are used such as cognitive behavioural strategies, exercises to help you let go of lingering resentments, word usage exercises and relaxation techniques. Building on a combination of ideas, the author has created an integrated course of action to help improve your existing anger management skills. This book provides tried and tested evidence-based strategies to help equip those who desire to make changes in how they react in angry and stressful situations.

This Book highlights:

The Impact of Anger on our Bodies

Clear Strategies for Preventing Anger Outbursts

How to process and Manage Lingering Resentments

How to Become Self - Reflective and Assertive

About the author

Mark Chapman is a London based Clinical Psychologist, licensed with two Professional Bodies, the South African Health Council Professional Board and the British Psychological Society. Mark presents keynote addresses, and conducts workshops with educators and people in business. Mark completed Post Graduate research at the Nelson Mandela Metropolitan University. He provides psychological insets for organizations and runs anger management groups and workshops across South Africa, United Kingdom and Europe. Mark's area of special interest is in group work, where he has successfully run Anger Management Groups, Self-Esteem Groups, Stress-Management Groups, and Depression-Support Groups both within a clinical and industrial environment. After years of clinical multidisciplinary reflection and an extensive review of his practical work, Mark has completed this life skills anger management-working book to complement the seven-week course he offers.

Mark can be reached by email: markchapman_psy@yahoo.com

Corporate and Individual Anger Management Clinics available upon request

'**Discover the Roots to Your Anger**' consists of combined interventions, which integrate cognitive behavioural interventions, communication skills, cognitive reflection and relaxation techniques. Practical strategies are cited and parts of this work originate from the author's own clinical psychology training.

Examples are shared from the author's experience working in a multidisciplinary team and clinical practice both in South Africa and London, UK.

The treatment models used are flexible and accommodate racial, cultural and gender issues.

Emphasis is placed on teaching one to identify the source and roots of anger, recognizing the cues and developing cognitive behavioural strategies to deal more effectively with anger.

Mark D Chapman

Licensed and Registered Chartered Clinical Psychologist with the British Psychological Society - United Kingdom & Registered for Independent Clinical Practice with the Health Councils Profession of South Africa.

Email: markchapman_psy@yahoo.com

Publishers Note

This publication is designed to provide accurate and authoritative information in regards to the effective management of anger. This work however, is no substitute for thorough professional training and is advised that adherence to ethical and legal standards is maintained. The health care professional at a minimum should be:

- Qualified and licensed to practice the profession of psychology with the relevant registration bodies.

- The professional must not "guarantee" a specific outcome.

Table of Contents

Suggested Course Structure xxi

Introduction 1

Principles and Theoretical Framework 4

Skills based 5

Anger and its impact on your physical health and relationships 5

Self-assessment 6

Self-Assessment Questions 7

Self-realization 8

Defence Mechanisms 8

Course Content 9

Course Objectives 11

Prerequisites 11

Process of Anger Management 12

Group Work 13

Causes and Results 14

Imitation 15

Punishment 15

Aggressive Impulses and Frustration 16

Self-Sabotage 18

The Characteristics of Passive Anger 18

Anger Control Plan and Timeouts 26

Toolbox & Control Plan Example: 28

Anger and the Family 29

Cognitive Behavioural Treatments 31

A - B - C – D Model And Thought Stopping 33

Should System 35

Irrational Beliefs / Faulty Thinking Patterns 37

Verbally abusive relationships 40

Thoughts - Words - Beliefs - Behaviour - Results 42

Underlying Emotions and Resentments 43

Resentment 44

Forgiveness 47

Communication skills and mind skills 55

Calming Phase and Deep Breathing 55

Music 57

Techniques And Strategies 59

Summary - Note from the Author 65

Two frogs fell into a can of milk,

Or so I've heard it told;

The sides of the can were shiny and steep

The milk was deep and cold.

"oh, what's the use?" croaked Number One,

"Tis fate; no help's around."

"Goodbye, my friend! Goodbye, sad world!"

And weeping still he drowned,

But Number two, of sterner stuff,

Dog-paddled in surprise,

The while he wiped his milky face and dried his milky eyes.

"I'll swim a while at least," he said - Or so I've heard he said.

"It really wouldn't help the world if one more frog was dead."

An hour or two he kicked and swam,

Not once he stopped to mutter,

Then hopped out, via butter!

- T.C. Hamlet

SUGGESTED COURSE STRUCTURE

WEEK ONE
Introduction to Anger Management
Principal & Theoretical Framework
Course Content & Self – Assessment

WEEK TWO
Course Objectives
Victim Anger; Imitation; Punishment;
Aggressive Impulses & Frustration
Self - Sabotage; Passive - Aggression

WEEK THREE
Cognitive Behavioural Approaches to Anger Management
Anger Control Plans; Timeouts
Anger & the Family Exercise
A-B-C-D Model for Anger Management

WEEK FOUR
'Should System' of Thinking
Cognitive Restructuring Exercise
Verbally Abusive Relationships; Word Technique
Underlying Emotions & Resentment

WEEK FIVE
Letting go of Resentment
Forgiveness Inventory (EFI)
Communication and Mind Skills

WEEK SIX
Techniques & Strategies
Calming Phase & Relaxation Skills

WEEK SEVEN
Summary & Feedback Session

INTRODUCTION

Anger is one of our most dynamic and forceful emotions moving us very powerfully. Emotions are not good or bad; they are simply part of life. What we choose to do with these emotions indicates whether they become positive or negative. If angry feelings are suppressed they may never become recognized or named. This could lead to mental health problems. Anger turned inwards is the cause of many relationship problems. Anger may trigger anxiety. Anxiety may in turn produce anger. Just because you are angry does not necessarily imply that you have a problem. Anger is after all, part of a natural response that aids in our survival and helps us to protect others.

Anger, can therefore give one the courage to protect our loved ones; it may warn others not to take advantage of us and in some instances confirm our own individuality. Anger can also be a healthy emotion, as it can lead us to take appropriate action. Anger can also help us to '*make right the wrongs*' in our lives and to face up to our personal issues. Facing up to your anger can also lead to the contribution of positive self-esteem and enhanced feelings of self-worth.

Anger does not always lead to devastating circumstances. However, left untreated, it can lead to psychological problems or can actually '*exacerbate*' existing ones. As medical intervention can be an effective antidote for infectious diseases, similarly applying anger management strategies can be an effective antidote to dysfunctional anger and recurring resentments. Serious physical wounds need serious medicine and require the skill of a physician to detect the source of the problem. Serious deep-rooted anger also requires the attention and skill of a health care professional.

Many people have found that anger can be a difficult emotion to manage. People often confuse anger with aggression. Aggressive behaviour is intended to cause harm to another person or property. This type of behaviour includes verbal threats or acts of physical abuse. Anger is an emotion that does not always lead to aggression. Therefore a person can still be angry without acting aggressively. The instinctive, natural way to express anger is to respond aggressively. A degree of anger as stated is necessary to our survival. However, we can't physically lash out at every person or object that annoys or irritates us. We need to find a balance between our angry feelings and finding practical ways of processing and managing these feelings in a constructive way.

Some people allow their anger to settle into lifelong resentments that have the potential to ultimately destroy or rob them of leading a successful life. Anger and lingering resentments can trap a person in a cycle of negative thinking, self justification, shame and guilt. Shame is actually the fear of what others will think of us if they ever find out what has happened to us or if they find out how we have reacted in certain situations. Guilt, on the other hand, is how we feel about ourselves as a result of violating our own internal standards that we have set for ourselves. When we become excessively angry or overreact in situations, we can be left feeling guilty, frustrated or shameful.

If you can't get on with people as a result of your angry and defensive outlook, then it becomes difficult to get on with 'life' itself. Some of the greatest pleasures in life involve relationships with other people. People help us experience the highs and lows of life. Learning anger management skills and relationship skills is a choice that anyone can make. An important question to ask is '**Do I want to get on with people?**'

Most people would agree that they want to be liked and accepted for who they are. If a person is holding on to deep-seated anger and lingering resentments it can be very difficult for others to tolerate and accept them. Generally people that are successful in relationships share some common characteristics, such as having a measure of compassion towards others, being able to show respect and being able to manage difficult emotions. Good interpersonal relationships include the ability to manage anger successfully. It is evident that improving relationships with others starts with oneself. One of the keys to making changes is in accepting that you need to modify certain parts of yourself.

One of the most important changes is in improving your own set of emotional management skills. We tend to see others as we see '*ourselves*' and we often dislike in others what we dislike in '*ourselves.*' If we have deep-seated anger and lingering resentments, then we tend to attract others with similar problems to ourselves. In most relationships, angry people tend to feel insecure, interpreting the world around them based on their feelings. High levels of self-interest and an aggressive outlook can destroy relationships. Becoming more aware of our anger and how it can impact our relationships is a crucial stage in making the required change.

The most important aspect in the process of change is learning the skill of being self-reflective with your anger, and less self-focused. Taking a mature sense of responsibility towards making the changes is vital to success. When you decide to accept responsibility, make the choice to change and apply some of the principles in this book, you may begin to notice that some of your relationships start to change for the better. Anger starts becoming a problem when it is felt too intensely, too frequently, or is expressed inappropriately. Even if your anger does not result in violence, the inappropriate expressions of aggressive outbursts almost always result in negative consequences. A consequence of these outbursts may be that people develop a fear of you; they may loose respect for you and even alienate you from their social circles.

This book is organized to reflect a therapeutic process that incorporates various levels and stages of anger management and contains a therapeutic intervention with a specific focus on understanding the source of your anger and resentment. Cognitive behavioural techniques help identify and restructure *'thinking patterns'* that precipitate anger. Principles to motivate and expand awareness are used throughout. There is a therapeutic sequence in mind, which can be used most effectively if the process is followed carefully. The book begins with a description of anger and its impact on our behavior, reviewing the process of anger, its source, impact and outcomes. Passive-aggression is covered in more detail and practical examples have been cited throughout the book which will help you find the source and roots of your anger, identify lingering resentments, and finally provide evidence-based strategies to help change faulty thinking patterns.

People often ask, *'How long will this process take?'* This is a difficult question to answer. We are all unique individuals and psychological growth and self-awareness levels differ. However, it is certain that the more able you are to self-reflect and share your *'struggles'* with others, the more likely the process of change will accelerate. The book covers problem-solving information that provides and equips the reader with sufficient skills to manage anger in a productive way. Anger management treatment is a complex process often requiring a multidimensional perspective.

Principles and Theoretical Framework

The theoretical framework incorporated in this book draws on Novaco (1975) and his work, which explores a cognitive behavioural conceptualization of anger. This theory identifies anger as a reaction to a *'perceived threat'*, in that the cognitive, behavioural and physiological responses are areas of potential change. According to research (Edmondson & Conger, 1996; Trafate, 1995; Williams, 2001; Department of Health, 2001), it can be assumed that the average participant undergoing a cognitive behavioural therapy intervention for the reduction of anger, generally improved in learning new anger management skills. These results appear consistent with other research that explored the effectiveness of cognitive behavioural interventions in the treatment of depression (Dobson, 1989) and anger (Van Balkom et al., 1994). Positive anger management strategies usually take place in two distinct phases: the first attempting to address the *'source of the anger,'* the second teaching participants *'coping skills'* (Novaco, 1975).

Skills based

Anger is a growing problem around the world. This is an emotion that most people feel frequently and strongly. Anger in relationships is widespread and can interfere with personal satisfaction and happiness. Ultimate success in life is closely associated with how well one manages difficult emotions. Despite this fact most people receive little, if any, *'systemic skills-based training in anger management.'* Anger management skills are important in the process of building good social relationships. Coping skills and adaptive resources are required for managing anger effectively.

Anger and its impact on your physical health and relationships

There is a large body of evidence suggesting a relationship between anger and one's physical health. When we are angry, our bodies react by producing stress-fighting responses in the nervous and endocrine systems. However, if these reactions continue over time it can become too much and the body begins to break down. Feeling anger too intensely or frequently places extreme 'stress' on the entire body. During long episodes of anger, certain parts of the nervous system become highly activated. The physical effects of anger can increase adrenalin surges, consequently having a negative impact on the body. Medical research and psychological theory have long since recognized that chronic hostility and anger, whether suppressed or vented, can be strong causative factors in depression, headaches, heart problems, high blood pressure, insomnia, intestinal disorders and ulcers (Huang, 1990).

Mismanaged anger is one of the major causes of conflict in our personal and professional relationships. Are you tired of allowing your anger to cripple you by holding grudges against people, by self-punishment, self-sabotage and destructive thoughts? If so, please read on! This course may be for you. If you are angry with someone else, you allow him or her to live *'rent-free in your mind.'* Are you having difficulty forgiving someone for something they did or did not do? Did someone make a mistake that you can't forget? If you are angry with another person for any reason, you allow them to *'control'* you. What events, people or resentments are you carrying or holding onto that are making you unhappy?

Self-assessment

You will be required to complete an Enright Forgiveness Inventory (EFI) and psycho-metric measures to assess your individual strengths and difficulties. This will ensure that an accurate qualitative measurement of interpersonal functioning in the affective, behavioural and cognitive domains is assessed (Subkoviak, Enright et al., 1992).

Discover the Roots to Your Anger

You will also be required to complete an Inventory Form so that specific changes can be *'measured, compared and scored.'* During the process of self-assessment you will be required to answer certain questions related to your own personal anger, and begin to think about the following:

Self-Assessment Questions

- *Do you find it increasingly difficult to 'trust' others at school, in the work place or at home?*

- *Do thoughts and fear of 'loneliness' keep holding you back from getting on with your life?*

- *Have you caught yourself being overly concerned with what others 'think' of you at work or college?*

- *When things don't work the way you want, do you tend to think to yourself, 'What have I done this time?'*

- *Are there times when you feel that the world and people are 'against' you no matter what you do?*

- *Do you become 'sad and anxious' for no reason then, all of sudden, you have an anger outburst, ending up feeling intensely guilty?*

- *Do you always want to keep the 'peace' at all costs, shying away from confrontation?*

If you agree with some of these questions, there may be a high probability that you have unresolved anger that could have kept you from reaching your *'full potential'* in some way. Finding out the 'root causes' of your anger can help you reach new levels of personal freedom, providing valuable insights into managing uncomfortable emotions. In order to uncover the source of your anger you need to be willing to examine your personal levels of anger and be prepared to engage in the often painful process of self-reflection. It is vital for you to start asking yourself the question, *'How have I contributed to this aggressive situation, could I have reacted differently?'*

Self-realization

The chances are high that if you do have a problem with anger you already know it and are aware of some of its *'roots'*. If you find yourself acting in ways that seem out of control and frightening, this anger management course may be for you. The process involves uncovering the source of your anger and becoming more aware of the depth and level of this emotion. The course is designed to increase your own self-awareness and self-reflective skills.

You will be required to follow specific exercises to help you become more aware of your anger. These exercises have been carefully selected for their individual validity and potential to help with the often painful process of self-reflection and self-awareness. All the exercises are *'evidence-based'* and have been used very successfully on *'advanced anger management'* workshops over the years.

Defence Mechanisms

As you progress on the course, you may find out that your anger may have been blocking out underlying emotions and feelings such as shame and guilt. At some stage you may also feel that you have been terrified of these aggressive feelings and have not allowed yourself to process them. Some people use defence mechanisms to protect themselves against difficult emotions. Common defence mechanisms that people use are denial, suppression, displacement and over-identification with the person that has harmed you. The course is designed to help you identify any *'defence mechanisms'* you are using to protect yourself from confronting the hurt and psychological *'pain'* in your life.

Some of these defence mechanisms help and serve to protect you from the psychological pain caused by lingering resentments. During the course you may be required to muster up the psychological resources to confront your anger and frustration in practical ways. Sometimes we are not able to muster up these resources on our own. However, there comes a point when we all need to deal with some of these defences in positive and constructive ways. By attending the anger management course you are taking action and responsibility for your feelings and personal responsibility for your angry reactions or behaviour.

Course Content

The course also consists of relaxation techniques, cognitive behavioral therapy, and rational-emotive-therapy. Offering specific strategies to change or modify angry feelings, thoughts and emotions. Specialized strategies are shared to help you deal with recurring resentments. As previously stated, the theoretical framework draws on Novaco's (1975) *'cognitive behavioural conceptualization of anger.'* This framework views anger as a reaction to a perceived threat in which the cognitive, behavioural and physiological responses are examined closely and carefully.

In terms of the relaxation techniques, it is assumed that anger and relaxation are learned behaviours. The theoretical framework draws on *'social learning theory'* as its premise for changes in behaviour. In other words, it's not possible to be angry and relaxed at the same time. During the relaxation stage, specific breathing exercises and muscle relaxation techniques are introduced.

The course is based on the assumption that our *'thoughts'* are the primary cause of angry emotions. If we can learn to recognize angry thoughts, we can stop *'angry feelings.'* A series of cognitive behavioral exercises are recommended as part of the process of managing anger. During the course you will be required to keep a log of the various forms of your anger and its intensity in different *'environments.'* The recording process helps to identify definite patterns relating to your anger outbursts.

During the course participants are encouraged to test out new ways of communicating with others. Strategies implemented are also drawn from Ellis (1977), using his work with anger management which is approached from a rational-emotive perspective. Ellis (1977) notes that our resentments are caused by *'unreasonable demands that all people must treat us with absolute fairness.'* In his work Ellis (1977) contends that it is possible to change unrealistic expectations so that we no longer expect others to be perfect. The model of work is based on the assumption that anger is essentially an irrational response.

Improved ways to respond and react will be introduced throughout the course, to help change specific perceptions that in the past have caused you to react in an angry or aggressive way. The latter part of the course includes helping you identify the source of your anger, which focuses on examining deep-seated resentments towards those that have hurt you in the past. You will be helped to reflect on the source and extent of your anger within a *'family perspective,'* using a set of questions.

Course Objectives

This course is designed to help you in the following areas:

- *You will be encouraged to examine your own thinking and own anger management skills in a safe structured environment.*

- *To help you to see an anger outburst as an opportunity to convert self-contempt into self-respect.*

- *To teach you ways to respect yourself.*

- *To identify irrational belief systems.*

- *To help you understand the role negative attitudes have in the rehabilitative and regenerative process.*

- *To help you improve your relationships skills.*

- *To apply evidence-based recognized anger management techniques.*

Prerequisites

Chronic anger is almost always accompanied by uncomfortable emotional and painful feelings. It is vital to the success of this course to refrain from '*blaming others*' for your pain, anger and dissatisfaction with life. As stated, healthy constructive anger management involves taking '*full responsibility*'. Blaming others for one's anger does not lead to healthy developmental skills and will not promote self-reflection and '*emotional empowerment.*'

Being open-minded is another necessary skill to develop. Tolerance and being open-minded is an important part of anger management (Williams & Williams, 1993). An open mind helps one to assess if the situation is important enough to pursue, compromise, or simply ignore. Some people are not able to *'listen'* to others and become *'intolerant'* to the views of others. On the other hand, open-minded people are continually *'growing and learning'* new ways to respond. During this course you will have the opportunity of allowing other participants the chance to offer their views and *'solutions'* on some of the angry situations people find themselves in. Essentially you will need:

- A desire to address your anger in 'practical' ways.

- To have the willingness and capacity to undergo continual 'self-examination.'

- A desire to 'avoid' the pain of the consequences of anger.

Process of Anger Management

The course is designed to help you change patterns of thinking by:

- Helping you to recognize damaging patterns of thoughts and behaviours as 'cognitive distortions.'

- Helping you learn new ways to process and 'order your thoughts'.

- Teaching you to respond in constructive ways to anger rather than 'destructive' ways.

- The application of 'practical strategies' to overcome anger.

Group Work

Many people perform tasks better when in the presence of others than alone. Groups can build social competence, foster empathy and responsiveness and develop a sense of belonging. This process can be referred to as *'social facilitation,'* and often occurs in many different environments. Agreement to attend this anger management course is therefore indicating that your desire for change with others is *'strong'* otherwise you would not have been interested in making the changes in the first place. People in groups tend to work harder and seem much more committed to change. This interesting phenomenon regarding performance in groups is not confined to people; this occurs in the ant population as well. Chen (1937) compared the amount of sand dug by ants when they were alone or in pairs or in a group of three. He found that groups of two and three did not differ appreciably, but in both conditions the ants dug more than three times as much sand per ant as they did when they were alone.

A group-based anger management strategy is one way to address anger control issues; however the final decision should be based on an *'assessment'* of individual circumstances. Some people find it difficult to relate in a group preferring to work on anger issues in *'individual anger management sessions.'* This anger management course can be delivered in a group setting or individually. The ideal number of participants is 15. There is sufficient empirical evidence to support group cognitive-behavioral interventions (Maude-Griffin et al., 1998; Smokowski & Wodarski, 1996; Yalom, 1995). Heimberg (1994) indicates that groups also provide a wider range of *'behavioural rehearsal activities.'* The anger management course is presented in a structured and safe environment, managed by a *'licensed'* and Chartered Clinical Psychologist.

Victim Anger

Sometimes we are aware of our anger and by repetition we keep leading ourselves into trouble over and over again. We then become despondent and feel that we are in a trap, resulting in becoming a *'victim of our own anger.'* Sometimes we develop a need to *'show'* the world how wrong it has been towards us, as we manifest a form of victim anger. Victim anger can strike at our identity and self-worth ultimately leading to an unhappy existence. When we become a victim of our own anger we become helpless, frustrated, and often feel hopeless.

Causes and Results

Feelings of anger can also be caused by death, divorce, abuse, families who purposefully withhold affection, feuding families, people making up cowardly slander against you, a boss or teacher who treats you with disdain and rejection, or nations that are at constant war. All these feelings and situations can also cause major health problems. Excessive anger can also be caused by health problems, drug or alcohol abuse, financial problems, performance related stress and anxiety at work or college.

Anger can also result from the intellectual frustration of knowing that your story has not been heard or that others are simply missing the point. Anger can also be the confused experience of childhood hurt and pain that has never been processed. Have you ever seen a child, hurt by something said or done, screaming out, "I hate you," "I wish you were dead!" Following this the child storms out of the room and cries uncontrollably. After a while the tears dry and all is forgotten. Nothing is said about the words used in this tantrum and life goes on as usual. If left unprocessed, some of these words can get forgotten into the back of the mind, collecting cobwebs of guilt and deep inner-resentment or anger.

Imitation

Young people at home and adults in the work place do not imitate indiscriminately; they imitate some people more than others. The more important, powerful, successful and liked people are, the more likely they are to be imitated. Most people have a strong tendency to imitate others; this imitation extends to virtually every kind of behaviour including aggression and anger. A young person observes parents being aggressive or even them controlling their aggression and albeit they tend to *'copy'* what they see. In many cases our own anger is shaped and determined by what we have observed as a child. If a child observes his or her parents, behaving with self-discipline, respect, dignity and a 'capacity to order their lives,' there is a good chance that the child will learn that this is the way to live life.

Punishment

A young person depends on his or her parents or caregiver for *'reinforcement'* and imitation. This can produce an interesting consequence. Punishing a young person for acting aggressively may be considered an effective method of teaching non-aggression, but may well produce the opposite effect. Punishment it seems should make the aggressive behaviour less likely in the future. The young person learns that they will be punished if they hit others, so to avoid punishment the aggressive behavior towards others is reduced.

A young person who is punished for fighting does tend to be less aggressive. However, a child who is *'punished severely'* for being aggressive at home tends to be more aggressive and angry than does a child who is punished less severely (Sears, Whiting, Nowlis, & Sears, 1953). According to this explanation the child will tend to imitate their parents or caregiver's aggressive behaviour. When the child has the upper hand, they tend to act the way their parents do towards them. The parents are *'aggressive'* and so is the child.

It appears that punishment can teach the child not to be aggressive at home, but it can also teach that aggression is acceptable *'if'* they can get away with it. Regardless of what the parents' are hoping for, children will continue to do what their parents do as well as what they say. If a parent models calm, relaxed behaviour the chances are high that the young person will follow this role. Parents who are open about their negative feelings and manage these challenges in front of their children, model positive ways in dealing with anger. If parents demonstrate good anger management skills, the chances are high that these important areas may be transferred to the child observing.

Aggressive Impulses and Frustration

An aggressive impulse or feeling is an internal state that cannot be easily observed directly. One can certainly see facial expressions or other physical signs when people are angry. However, angry feelings may not be that easy to identify in others. Anger can also be expressed indirectly, when some situations or persons can leave you feeling tense and very frustrated. If you are not aware of the roots and source of these feelings it could lead to one manoeuvering innocent people into conflict. As a result of your anger, you may have the additional struggle of trying to process the 'lingering' resentments which are caused by your internal strife.

We all experience anger; virtually everyone at one time or another has experienced revengeful feelings towards others. Some of these feelings are not necessarily expressed openly. Aggressive impulses can be studied by asking how one is feeling in certain anger provoking situations, as a reasonably reliable indicator. When we are bothered or hurt by someone, we can feel aggressive towards the person or situation. Such as the reaction of a driver who is waiting for a traffic light to change from red to green, and, before it does, the driver of the car behind starts 'blowing their horn'. As a result, depending on how the injured person perceives this they may react with anger and possibly aggression. Psychological reactions to being hurt or frustrated can lead to feelings of 'indignation and animosity' towards the offender or offending situation. These feelings and thoughts can manifest in actions such as screaming, throwing a temper tantrum or behaving in an irrational way. In more severe cases this can lead to road rage and physical assault.

Frustration, on the other hand, is the interference with or blocking of goal attainment. If people's goals are blocked by certain situations we may experience aggressive feelings. Depending how these uncomfortable feelings are 'managed,' determines the eventual outcome. The issue is that the victim perceives the frustration or attack as intended harm if it instigates anger or aggressive behavior. That is, the victim arrives at the conclusion that his or her tormentor intended to frustrate or annoy them.

We all feel irritated when someone or something obstructs our needs or desires. However, there is a clear distinction between anger and feeling hurt or irritated. Anger separates itself in that its desire is 'to get even' with someone that has hurt or harmed you. Revenge is sought. This revenge can also be an 'unconscious' part of us that we are not aware of unless brought to the 'conscious.' With the aid of a series of practical exercises you will be helped to bring some of your unconscious anger to your conscious. Again, this process may enhance your self-reflection skills, and could set you on a path of leading a successfully 'managed' lifestyle, relatively free from destructive anger outbursts.

Self-Sabotage

We have internalized many of the standards and expectations of others and at times find ourselves comparing ourselves with others. We can often end up in a process of 'self-punishment.' If we have a strong urge to seek revenge and do not take action, we can sometimes turn these destructive feelings on ourselves as a form of self-sabotage. In some cases we hope that our self-inflicted suffering will get the message across to others such as 'Look what you made me do to myself.' The cycle can also be repeated over and over again, unless one takes the steps to make the changes and shifts in perceptions that are required. Our self-sabotage could then move into a self-blaming mode. For example, we end up continually apologizing to people at the most 'inappropriate times.' This in turn leads to further self-criticism, all of which stems from unresolved, unprocessed deep-rooted anger.

The Characteristics of Passive Anger

Description

Passive-aggression often occurs when an individual is requested to do something that they don't wish to do. By simply 'appearing' to agree, without making a firm commitment, they can avoid the request. Levels of passive-aggression differ. The more extreme forms are when people agree to do something about the request and then fail to carry out their agreement.

Passive-aggression is often a method used by family or subordinates who are unable to oppose their superiors. As a result they turn to subtle and indirect means to communicate anger and aggression. Passive-aggression can be rooted in a 'difficult childhood,' where a helpless child or teenager is not able to protect themselves from abusive parents or authority figures. Instead of managing this painful issue some young people simply don't have the skills to deal with this and in their frustration resort to turning their anger inwards.

There are a host of behaviours that are seemingly passive in nature although in fact they are actually overtly aggressive expressions. Holding on to resentments, which are then expressed behind people's backs or in unnecessary comments in conversations, are all examples of passive aggression. In the work place we often agree about something but never 'follow through' with it as in fact we do not really agree with it. One may also agree at all costs with those in authority and then procrastinate, ending up never doing what was promised in the first place.

Roots of passive-aggression

Passive-aggression can stem from 'modeling' passive-aggressive parents. The child learns that the only way to behave and survive at home is to become passively aggressive themselves. Alternatively this could also be learnt from acting in the 'opposite' way to a violent parent or caregiver.

Passive-aggressive behaviour can also stem from repressed anger. In some cases it may be a symptom of deeper issues like co-dependency, acute anxiety and possibly clinical depression.

Interpersonal Relationships

Other people will easily notice your behaviour and react in various ways. Often those who act in a passive-aggressive way will eventually become disappointed in you. This can cause lots of unhelpful misunderstandings as people find out that you have not been 'consistent' in what you have said. People often become resentful and mistrusting of each other as a result. Sometimes a passive-aggressive individual will act out 'annoying behaviour' that they are completely unaware of. The impact this behaviour has on others can destroy relationships. Those that are passive- aggressive find it extremely difficult to practice 'self-discipline' and are often oblivious of how this could cause conflicts in relationships.

Sometimes the passive-aggressive individual has a desire to 'keep the peace' at all costs. It can be so potent that they avoid any form of confrontation, deceiving themselves that they will never win anyway, so what is the point in trying? Others believe that they are not 'winners,' and never challenge topics. People with this irrational belief system usually feel they are without hope or that no substantial changes will ever take place in their lives so why bother trying.

Cognitive Behavioral Approaches and Passive-Aggression

There are, however, certain irrational thinking patterns that seem to support passive-aggression. This may start with one erroneous idea or thought about others, such as 'Nobody cares how I feel,' 'No one will ever understand my true feelings.' Others may feel that they need to conceal their true feelings. Faulty thinking patterns such as these can have a 'negative impact' on relationships.

As a result of this faulty thinking, people spend much of their time hiding these aggressive feelings and thoughts. In turn this can lead to backing down to avoid conflict at all costs. True feelings are hidden rather than openly expressing them. Hiding angry feelings is a classic example of passive-aggression. Usually the person will hide their feelings of anger, as they are terrified that if they disagree on a topic, the consequence will result in some form of 'rejection.' The passive-aggressive person thinks that it's better to deny feelings, so as to avoid the risk of 'upsetting' others. Often the passive-aggressive individual ends up lying about how they truly feel and think in a futile attempt to keep the peace.

Indications of Passive-Aggressive Behaviour

It is important for you to understand and recognize when a person acts passively aggressive towards you. This section will highlight some of the 'signs' that can help you identify more clearly when this happens.
Perhaps the first indication is when a person at work, school or in a social context keeps on 'agreeing' with what you are saying, even if you are being rigid in your thinking. People who never dare to disagree with your perceptions and views tend not to talk at all about 'negative feelings' avoiding any hint of disagreement with you. Unpleasant topics are invariably avoided at all costs in order to avoid potential clashes. When you approach passive-aggressive individuals with an uncomfortable topic, they tend to react by withdrawing or being silent. Reactions like these may indicate that someone is passively-aggressive towards you.

Another clear indication that someone is passively-aggressive towards you is when he or she makes no effort at all to try and 'improve' your relationship with them. They tend to talk irrationally about problems in the relationship or even deny that there is a problem. These people often engage in 'magical thinking' about how they are going to make changes in their lives, what solutions they have thought of, and then fail to carry out these plans. Some may revert to patronization as a defence tool in difficult situations. Others may minimize problems, trying to make you believe that you are 'imagining' the whole process. There may also be ongoing denial that there is a problem in the relationship despite the clear evidence that exists.

List of Passive-Aggressive Behaviours:

- *Talking behind people's backs; using cowardly slander against others.*

- *Listening to gossip: spreading rumors about others.*

- *Using the 'silent treatment.'*

- *Not maintaining good eye contact. Looking at a person's forehead instead of their eyes in an attempt to avoid eye contact.*

- *Living out your pain or frustrations in others. Projecting 'negative moods' onto others.*

- *Displaying facial expressions such as sour face or a sulking demeanour.*

- *Provoking other people into an aggressive role, and then offering 'patronizing forgiveness.'*

- *Encouraging aggression in others and as soon as there is a response, backing down and trying to remain neutral.*

- *Using emotional blackmail.*

- *Not showing any signs of anger, but crying instead, usually with a helpless tone.*

- *Finding all sorts of medical complaints to gets one's own way, or in an attempt to make others feel guilty.*

- *Sabotaging relationships by never being on time, forgetting the venues that were arranged, turning up a few hours late and then expecting people not to be unhappy about it.*

- *Using a partner, friend, or child to convey negative feelings of some sort to someone that you are angry with.*

- *Holding back love and affection, withholding deserved*

Discover the Roots to Your Anger

compliments and consciously deciding not to show any positive feelings towards others.

- *Trying to please others in any shape or form possible; becoming so self sacrificing and overly helpful in any situation despite how you feel.*

- *Always making do with hand-me-downs or second best, being afraid to tell others that you are not prepared to accept second best anymore.*

- *Knowingly destroying relationships between people. Purposefully and intentionally leaving people out of events and invitations for social gatherings.*

- *Making drawn-out, suffering sighs and refusing to get involved with a requested activity; leaving all the responsibility in the hands of other people.*

- *Making unfriendly comments or rude sarcastic comments when they are not forthcoming.*

- *Unconsciously and consciously setting up plans and social arrangements that you know will fail, for example, inviting people that you know have a personality clash, to a social gathering.*

- *Never learning from past mistakes and failures.*

- *Always under-achieving, never putting any effort into anything. This includes schoolwork, in the workplace, on the sports field and also in relationships. Always seeing yourself as an underachiever and a victim of circumstance, not willing to take responsibility for choices made.*

- *Highlighting and expressing frustrations about minor issues and consciously avoiding or intentionally not noticing the major ones.*

- *Non-verbal behaviour could include giving someone the 'cold shoulder,' an insincere smile, a limp handshake, a nasty or aggressive look, frowning at people, lifting your eyebrows,* shaking your head, sighing or staring at people.

- Making fatalistic statements about the world and offering no clarification for such statements. Often these negative statements are made in completely inappropriate environments.

- Speaking and intellectualizing about disappointments without showing any feelings at all.

The Characteristics of Aggressive Behaviour

- Threatening behaviour, frightening people by saying how you are going to physically hurt them.

- Finger pointing, leaning forward, hands on hips, fist shaking, and wearing symbols that are associated with violence.

- Purposefully driving behind someone at an unacceptable distance. Driving destructively and not bothering with the codes of practice on the roads.

- Opening cupboards in an aggressive fashion, clanging plates when washing up, throwing things around at home and slamming doors.

- Moving your legs up and down in an aggressive manner or tapping fingers. Pushing or shoving.

- Physical violence towards people or property, including writing on walls, buses and trains.

- Shouting at people; also verbally abusing them with dirty or humiliating remarks.

- Violating shared intimate feelings by telling others what was said to you in confidence.

- Deafening people with loud music and not bothering to consider *those around you.*

- *Overtly ignoring other people's feelings or ideas when they try and contribute to a discussion; cutting people short when they are trying to explain things.*

- *Making judgments about others, labeling people by putting them into a category.*

- *Knowingly polluting the environment with no sense of remorse for their actions. For example, leaving rubbish at a park for others to clean up.*

- *Bullying, such as using threats or violence to get weaker people to act against their will.*

- *Purposefully blinding oncoming traffic with full beam headlights because they have not dimmed their lights for you.*

- *Cutting in when driving or just switching from one lane to the other without consideration for others.*

- *Unjust blaming - accusing others of your own mistakes; blaming others for your own feelings of anger, using statements such as "You're getting me angry," "You drove me to it."*

- *Making unjust accusations, racial comments or general accusations about people or events.*

- *Intellectually abusing people; using sarcastic remarks, or speaking too fast, often intentionally a few steps ahead of the other person.*

- *Working too much, then expecting others to fit into your busy schedule*

- *Not considering the consequences of your actions, and the potential impact these actions could have on others.*

- *Expressing distrust in everyone, only willing to trust oneself.*

- *Not responding to other people's requests for assistance.*

- *Stopping any attempts to sort out frustrations. For example saying, "There is nothing I want to talk about."*

- *Refusing to forgive and forget past hurts.*

- *Intentionally doing something that will hurt another physically, emotionally or psychologically.*

- *Reacting unpredictably with mood swings, often without provocation.*

- *Explosive aggressive angry outbursts over minor issues.*

- *Attacking indiscriminately, often in an obtrusive manner.*

- *Using illogical arguments and saying "I don't care whether it makes sense or not."*

Anger Control Plan and Timeouts

It is important to develop a repertoire of anger management strategies, immediate strategies that may assist in a 'tense' situation. Some people prefer to use cognitive restructuring such as challenging hostile and negative self-talk or the self-analysis of core belief structures. Others prefer to use strategies such as thought-stopping or relaxation techniques. Having your own 'individualized anger management control plan' is very important and vital for the successful management of your anger. An anger management plan will help you record the anger-control techniques that work uniquely for you.

As you go through the various methods in this book, you can start recording and 'identifying strategies' that work for you, consciously referring to them in anger provoking situations. Some people call their anger control plans their 'toolbox' and refer to the individual strategies as 'tools.' The idea behind this process is that when you encounter an anger-provoking event, you have immediate access to your individualized anger control plan or 'toolbox.' The long-term objective of the anger management course is to develop a set of strategies that you can use for specific 'anger-invoking events' in your life. Throughout the course, a host of strategies are taught and additional strategies are summarized at the end of this book for ease of reference.

Timeouts

Timeout is a basic anger management strategy highly recommended for an 'anger control plan' or 'toolbox.' Timeout procedure is leaving the situation that is causing the escalation of anger. It is also stopping a conversation that you feel is provoking your anger. It is clear that a timeout plan needs to involve others. This involves an 'agreement' about a previously agreed plan and course of action. These agreed procedures may include family members, friends or colleagues at work. Any of the parties may at any time call a timeout in accordance with the rules that were agreed.

The person calling the timeout can leave the anger-provoking scene, if need be. In the agreement, the person leaving the situation may return to either finish the discussion or to postpone for a later date. Timeouts are excellent strategies to use in conjunction with other methods. For example, you can take a timeout and do some physical exercise by taking a long-refreshing walk in the park or at the beach.

TOOLBOX & CONTROL PLAN EXAMPLE:

MY ANGER MANAGEMENT CONTROL PLAN OR TOOLBOX

1. Take an Agreed Timeout

2. Share your feelings with others Strategies in this Book

3. Exercise Techniques

4. Use Relaxation Techniques

5. Challenge Irrational Thoughts

6. Eating Correctly

7. Refer to list of

8. Practice Breathing

9. Thought-Stopping

Anger and the Family

"I cannot think of any need in childhood as strong as the need for a father's protection." -Sigmund Freud 1856-1939, Austrian
Physician -Founder of Psychoanalysis

Growing up in an angry family environment can help in assessing one's own level of anger (Reilly & Grusznski, 1984). Interaction with aggressive parents can have an impact on one's ability to manage anger. It is important to note how past interactions with aggressive people especially relatives, could have an influence on current behaviour, thoughts, feelings and attitudes. Many people are unaware of the connections between past learning and current behaviour.

During this exercise, you will be encouraged to explore how your parents and other members of the family displayed anger and frustration. Basic patterns in relation to anger seem most prominent during the developmental process of our personalities. In our impressionable childhood years our basic personality is 'shaped and re-shaped.' For most people, the interactions with significant others such as parents have strongly influenced certain behaviours, thoughts, feeling and attitudes. Role models also play an important part in this process. The more important, powerful, successful and liked people are the more likely that they will be 'imitated.' Young people observe their parents being aggressive or observe them controlling their aggression, then generally tend to copy what they see.

During this exercise you will be asked a series of questions regarding your parents, families or caregivers. This exercise can provoke strong emotions and tends to be a highly sensitive topic.

If at any stage you feel uncomfortable answering questions, you do not have to do so. As there appears to be a natural tendency to elaborate on family issues because of the complexity of emotional content, you will be asked to keep to the questions asked. This exercise will take place in smaller working groups.

ANGER AND THE FAMILY (EXERCISE)

1. Write a brief description of your family.

2. Are there any family members that you don't get along with?

3. What kind of environment did you grow up in?

4. Can you describe how anger was dealt with in your family? Did your mother express anger differently from your father?

5. Did your family express positive emotions? If so how?

6. How were negative emotions expressed in your family?

7. Who used to discipline you and what methods were used?

8. Could you describe the role you played in your family?

9. Are there any behaviours, thoughts, feelings or negative attitudes that you have carried over from your growing up years?

Cognitive Behavioural Treatments

Cognitive behavioural therapy is now one of the leading techniques used to manage anger and clinical depression (Dyer, 2000). Cognitive behavioural therapy is also the most common form of psychological therapy used in the National Health Service today (Department of Health, 2001) and has proved successful in the treatment of chronic anger and its effective management (Ellis, 1993). This clinical approach focuses on helping its users understand the negative thought processes that can cause problems and attempts to restructure certain target thoughts so they become more balanced. Beck (1995) notes the important connection between thinking and anger management.

Often our negative thoughts can result from misinterpretation of events. We can often misunderstand the actions or motives of others. Beck (1995) argues that these faulty thinking patterns can include negative statements, such as 'I am not going to allow this person to walk all over me,' or 'who do they think they are?' Often these negative thoughts can lead to further anger outbursts and frustrations. In this course you will be taught to identify how your thoughts influence responses to anger provoking situations. Ellis (1993), a leading researcher in the field of anger management, notes that anger can be a result of a person's perception and can be managed by thinking a way out of unhealthy anger expressions.

Ellis (1993) places focus on helping individuals become aware of how thoughts, feelings and behaviour are closely related. Beck (1995) contends that emotions are influenced by a person's actual perception of an event. Following this explanation, sometimes it's not the event that causes the anger; it is what the person actually thinks about that causes the event (Beck 1995). The process of cognitive behavioural therapy helps in understanding how and why we act the way we do in certain situations. Using this approach we may gain insight into patterns of faulty thinking and negative perceptions. This will help in making the changes required. Tang (2001) completed an important retrospective study into the impact that cognitive behavioural therapy has on lowering the intensity of specific anger episodes. Tang (2001) found that cognitive behavioural therapy scores on the post treatment measures indicated a significant reduction in the group member's overall experience of intense anger, an improvement in cognitive behavioural coping styles and anger management skills.

This process can also be called cognitive restructuring. It can be a useful tool to stop negative thinking. It can help us put unhappy, negative thoughts 'under a microscope,' challenging them and discovering their root cause. This is vital to understand, as our negative thoughts in turn create negative moods. Negative moods reduce the quality of our interpersonal relationships and can potentially sabotage our social lives. The key point to understand is that **our moods are driven by what we tell ourselves.** The process of cognitive restructuring aids us in this process by evaluating how rational and valid our interpretations really are.

During this process you will be encouraged to learn positive responses to anger provoking situations. Strategies will be taught that help and encourage you to make respectful verbal and non-verbal responses. Schmidt (1993) notes that it is possible to tolerate uncomfortable feelings in a constructive way that is not harmful to one's self or to another person.

A - B - C – D

MODEL AND THOUGHT STOPPING

A = Activating Situation or Event.

B = Belief System - What you tell yourself about the
   event and your beliefs and expectations of others.

C = Consequence or outcome of events.

D = Dispute - Examination of certain beliefs and are they
   realistic or rational?

The A - B - C - D Model is part of a cognitive restructuring model, which was pioneered by Albert Ellis (Ellis 1979; Ellis & Harper, 1975). This process requires thought stopping as part of a strategy to overcome aggressive outbursts. Cognitive restructuring is an advanced anger management technique that demands self-reflection and the exact examination and identification of certain negative thoughts. Clearly, some participants may differ in their ability to learn and to apply some of these strategies, as success does depend on levels of motivation to change. Some people may not be ready to challenge their irrational beliefs. Whatever the person's level of readiness and openness to change, it is vital that skills are taught in an understandable format. The emphasis is on teaching how irrational beliefs perpetuate anger and the importance of modifying these beliefs to prevent further escalation of anger. During this phase the A - B – C – D model is discussed in depth, including the topic of thought-stopping. Regardless of how one views a particular belief as either irrational or maladaptive, most people recognize that some beliefs increase anger which could lead to aggressive behaviour (Ellis 1979; Ellis & Harper, 1975). Thought recognition and thought-stopping provide a direct strategy for helping people take control over specific beliefs that cause them to act aggressively.

Ellis (1979) describes A as the activating event. The activating event is the trigger that has caused the anger outburst. B represents the belief system that one has about the activating event. Ellis (1979) contends that it is not the events themselves that produce anger, but our interpretations of the specific belief about the event. C in this model represents the emotional consequence of the event. These are basically the feelings one experiences as a result of one's interpretations of and beliefs about the event. The A - B - C - D model consists of identifying beliefs that appear irrational and then taking the steps to dispute them. D in this model stands for 'dispute,' people who think that they should be in control of every situation are more prone to anger outbursts. It is clearly not possible to be in control of every situation, a better way to handle this could be to tell yourself that, 'I have no power over things that I can not control,' 'I have to start accepting the things that I really can't change, ' or 'There is nothing that I can do to bring back the past.' These are some examples of disputing beliefs that have caused problems with anger.

Beck (1995) notes that as people become angry, they engage in an internal dialogue, simply called 'self-talk.' Negative thoughts can sometimes result from misinterpretation of events and situations. An event or situation is basically misunderstood, largely due to an unhelpful belief system. Negative thoughts and self-talk can include statements such as 'I'll show you!' 'I am not going to let you get the best of me.' For example, a father's adolescent son says something rude to him. The father gets very angry with his son and shouts at him. He possibly would have much more success at managing his anger if he spoke to his son about how upset he is at being disrespected. In this case the father acted on his anger, which could have been avoided if he had the skills and knowledge to change his thinking.

Suppose you were at the post office in a long queue. As you approach the front of the queue people start pushing in front of you. In this situation you may start to get angry. You may be thinking, 'How can these people be so rude?' 'They have jumped the queue to try and get in first!' You may be thinking, 'These people just don't care about others.' Examples of irrational self-talk that can produce anger escalation are often reflected in statements such as 'People should be more considerate about my feelings,' 'How on earth can they be so inconsiderate and disrespectful to me?' 'These people just can't have been bothered about the rules of the post office' Ellis (1979) contends that people do not necessarily have to get angry when they encounter such events. Ellis (1993) notes that the event itself does not get them upset and angry; it is rather how people interpret the event and the underlying belief system concerning the event that causes anger.

Should System

People who struggle with managing their anger often have a well-developed 'should' system in place. A 'should' system is a person's values and expectations that are usually enforced or projected onto others. Ellis (1993) notes that imposing one's 'should' system onto others can potentially cause disastrous results, especially when others do not live up to one's values and expectations. These high expectations of others can lead to anger outbursts and unhelpful feelings. People generally do what they think they should do, as opposed to what others think they should do. Hence the potential for unmet expectations and possible conflicts in value systems may result. The 'should system' refers to all terminology that demands absolute adherence to beliefs and values. Clearly, if we adopt the 'should thinking' of other people and never examine them in terms of our own needs, we will most probably become angry and frustrated. Most people agree, for example, that showing respect to other people is an important quality. In reality, however, people do not respect each other in many different settings and situations. In this instance you can choose to view the situation more realistically, such as, 'All people have flaws and weaknesses.' 'You may ask yourself, if it's realistic to expect everyone you meet to respect you'.

On the other hand you could choose to let your anger escalate each time you witness, or are the recipient of, another's disrespect. Your belief system and perceptions regarding respect could keep you very angry, leading to anger and frustration. Holding this unhelpful belief could ironically lead you to show disrespect for others, which then in turn violates your own beliefs about how people should be respected. People have other irrational beliefs such as 'Everyone must respect what I do.' Holding such a rigid belief can cause anger, especially in the case when people reject you. By following the model and disputing this irrational belief, you could modify your self-talk by saying, 'Not all people are going to like me,' and 'I can't make people like me'; this may be enough to diffuse a potential anger outburst. Other irrational beliefs that are common are, 'I must be treated as an equal at all times.' By disputing this belief and saying to yourself, 'I cannot expect to be treated fairly by the entire community,' this self-statement in itself could in fact potentially reduce your anger and frustration rather significantly.

IRRATIONAL BELIEFS / FAULTY THINKING PATTERNS

All people must follow the rules of the road.

Life should be fair.

Good must always prevail over bad things in life.

People must do the right thing at all times.

I should never feel hurt or angry.

I should always be liked. People should not reject me.

I should like everyone I meet.

I must put the needs of others before my own.

I should know and anticipate all events in my life.

I must never make mistakes.

I should do everything perfectly.

Cognitive Restructuring (Exercise 1)

You will be asked to complete a 'cognitive restructuring table' and follow the process of cognitive or thought identification. You will be required to identify the events that make you angry. Write down the cues that were associated with the anger provoking event and the strategies used to manage anger in the previous week. Review the ABCD model and record at least two irrational beliefs. You will be asked how you managed to dispute some of these beliefs. The following points need to be included in the table:

Write down the situations that trigger your negative and angry thoughts.

Identify the moods that you felt in this situation.

Note the automatic thoughts you experienced when you felt the mood.

Look for evidence to support these negative thoughts.

Look for evidence that does not support these negative thoughts.

List the balanced thoughts you had in this situation.

Review in your diary and note your moods over the seven-week period, see if there are any changes.

Word - Technique (Exercise 2)

Words can be long lasting and have tremendous influence on our lives - some positive and others not so positive. The word session will help you identify any areas that have perhaps caused you pain in the past. Authentic attempts to put 'alternative strategies' in place will be discussed in a group format.

Urban (2004) notes that over many years people have a created a complex system of communication called language. With this system thousands of words have emerged. Words give meaning to our experiences. The first method of communication was with hands, pointing and making gestures, or using facial gestures. This, as we know, is called body language. According to Urban (2004), our ancestors wanted to communicate in more specific ways, so they started to draw pictures. The Egyptians created an advanced and complicated system of pictures known as Hieroglyphics. The term Hieroglyphics means 'pictorial characters.' It became clear that pictures and symbols were far more descriptive than hand signals. Now we have developed the ability to make associations between words and pictures.

Words have the power to transform our lives, psychologically and emotionally. Words influence our destiny. Words are able to create positive and negative emotions. Words used appropriately can motivate us, inspire us and help us achieve our goals. Words can also 'break us down' having the potential to cause all sorts of pain, hurt and anger. Words do have a lasting impact on us and often cause us to over 'react' in certain situations. In a more simple form, we use words to find meaning to our lives and also to indicate to others how we feel. Words are powerful, having a lasting impact.

Verbally abusive relationships

Verbally abusive relationships are rampant today. This may filter down from home to the workplace or school into the broader environment, sometimes into the global community. People often 'verbally abuse' each other; it's rather simple to conclude that this could be stemming from learned patterns in their environment or community. Young people and adults are often verbally threatened and this can turn into fear, submission or compliance. Ketterman (1992) notes that, 'Verbal abuse is any statement made to a victim that results in emotional damage.' 'Such damage can limit one's happiness and productivity and in some cases lasts a lifetime.' In essence, verbal abuse creates emotional wounds and scars that may permanently disfigure a person. Emotional scars and wounds, whilst leaving a permanent mark, can also serve a purpose: they can be reminders of the lessons we have learnt from painful experiences.

With words we can make critical judgements and can engage in harmful patterns of 'name-calling,' which is used to make someone feel 'less than' and it can lead to the victim becoming submissive to the perpetrator. Accusations, 'cowardly slander' and blaming others are all made up of words that can 'destroy' people. Sadly some of us have grown up in verbally abusive households and do not recognize verbal abuse in the middle of an angry discord with a partner or child. Passive behaviour or using words that undermine the other person are powerful forms of verbal abuse. Not saying what you mean, and then going behind someone's back to make things happen unbeknown to the other person is also verbally abusive and unfair.

Relationships are harmed by words that can demean the other individual. This usually results in a devalued relationship. In some cases this results in irretrievable differences, as we cannot take back what injury we have inflicted on others when we have said things in anger. Trying to take back words is like someone throwing a hand full of feathers into wind. It's impossible to recover all of the feathers. Once a negative word is spoken about another, whether true or false, it usually leaves a lasting impact. Similar forms of abuse fall under headings of 'forgetting' and 'withholding love.' By forgetting, this is a convenient way for the verbal abuser not to take responsibility. People who are verbally abusive usually feel little self-control over their own lives. Research also suggests that they have a lack of sense of self-worth and self esteem (Enright, 1998, Freedman, 1994, Subkoviak, 1992, Waters, 1984).

Word-Technique (Exercise 2 a)

This course highlights the power of words. Emphasis is placed on the ways we 'select' words. You will be asked to select words from two sets of lists and to make up sentences about them. The objective of this session is to illustrate that words, if used strategically, have a decided effect and 'impact' on us and other people. This word-technique is completed in smaller working groups.

The purpose of this word exercise is also to prepare you for easy identification of your own anger, and to start recognizing certain words that have managed to influence you. Some negative words that people may have said about you or spoken over you in the past may have intruded into your thinking patterns without you even being aware. The word techniques help us to uncover damaging words that people may have said to you in the past. Once uncovered, the process of bringing the 'unconscious' to the 'conscious' begins. During this exercise you will also be required to recall some of the 'positive,' 'constructive' words that have been spoken over you in your developing years. It is important for you to continue with journal entries to keep track of all the 'discoveries' that you are making.

Word-Technique (Exercise 2 b)

Understanding that anger, for the most part, begins with our thoughts and beliefs, is really the fundamental theme on this course. Initially we need to identify our own unique patterns of thoughts and self-talk. Then we need to examine our thoughts and underlying beliefs which are causing us to feel angry. As mentioned one of the keys to effective anger management is in understanding that we are unable to control 'every' potential anger-invoking event, regardless of where it comes from. What we can control is our 'reaction' to that specific stressor. Words, and their selection and correct choice can also be part of a unique reaction to stressors.

THOUGHTS - WORDS - BELIEFS - BEHAVIOUR - RESULTS

Take an example such as: 'People don't like me'. Holding onto a thought system like this, may run through one's mind on a consistent basis. As one thinks about this, certain words are used that support this thought. The phrase, 'People don't like me,' is repeated over and over, in one's self-talk and in discussion with others. This, in turn supports the initial belief that, 'People don't like me'. Our belief system, whether positive or negative, influences the way we behave and react. If one holds onto this belief system, we start acting accordingly. For example, one does not try and improve and change when we believe that people simply don't like us so what's the point in trying. The result is that we start to think *more* 'negative thoughts' and use associated words that 'reinforce' our belief system. During this exercise you will be asked to select a positive and negative belief about yourself in an anger-invoking situation. In the smaller working groups you will be encouraged to identify positive and negative words that reinforce your selection. The thoughts - words - beliefs - behaviour - and results process will be carefully examined in smaller working groups.

Underlying Emotions and Resentments

Anger can hide other primary emotions (Reilly, Clark, Shropshire, Lewis, & Sorensen, 1994). During the course you will be encouraged to reflect on some 'primary emotions' that have caused you difficulties in the past. Some of these hidden emotions are shame, hurt, feelings of powerlessness and loss of respect. It is important to try and identify some of the underlying feelings so that the primary emotions can be identified and dealt with more effectively. An example could be a worker who says something 'disrespectful' to his boss. This makes the boss angry, but the boss might have success in handling the issues in a positive way if he can get across to the worker that he is more concerned about the worker being disrespectful. If the boss acts on his anger, primary feelings get buried in the 'yelling and cursing.'

Resentment

The human mind is like a mountain: we only use that part of it that shows on the surface. The part that is evident is our conscious mind, that area that we have control over. However, beneath the mountain lays a 'deep foundation' and this represents the unconscious part of our minds. Within this lie strong feelings that have in some cases been 'repressed,' and sometimes these feelings do find expression in our lives in many complex ways. Hidden or repressed resentments can cause us to feel angry and frustrated. These feelings may go back many years, or may have been caused by recent hurts. Some people may feel that they have not received their just dues in life or have been unfairly treated in some way. Some people compare themselves with others and feel that they have not received as much love in their family as compared to others. Perhaps others feel that they deserve the promotion at work and have become resentful of others. All these disappointments and unmet expectations can lead to feelings of resentment.

Resentment expresses itself in all sorts of complex ways. Some people develop strong views about certain issues and are not afraid to tell others. Some people will manifest a rigid and hostile attitude upon an initial introduction. Others show 'rigid hostilities' toward groups of people. Deep-seated resentments can cause the greatest damage within the family circle. If an argument occurs or a family member becomes 'difficult to live with,' one can comfortably assume that the source of this problem may be some form of lingering resentment. Trying to overcome resentments is a complex task, requiring motivation and self-discipline to change.

During the process you will be required to examine when these feelings of resentment started. 'What caused these feelings? Once the source of your resentment is located, this may help in relieving difficult feelings and ultimately improve your relationships with others. You will be encouraged to learn ways to cope in future, so that you refuse to allow feelings of resentment to develop. This process if explained correctly enhances the understanding of the impact that your perceptions and underlying resentments have on anger. If you start to 'understand the process,' you will be better able to manage the underlying primary emotions such as hurt, shame, lingering resentments and loss of self-respect instead of relenting to your anger. You will be encouraged to practice underlying feeling identification in pseudo potential anger inducing situations, reporting back to your smaller work groups.

Practical Exercise - Resentment

Using practical exercises, the course is designed to help you change your perceptions regarding interpersonal forgiveness. As stated these involve the affective, behavioural and cognitive systems of the forgiver, and also feelings and emotions about the offender. During this process you will be required to complete an Enright Forgiveness Inventory (EFI). The Enright Forgiveness Inventory has been the measurement tool of choice in leading forgiveness research for the centre of Human Development studies at the University of Wisconsin. The EFI is an objective measure of the degree to which one person forgives another who has hurt him or her deeply and unfairly. The EFI consists of 60 items and three subscales composed of ten positive items and ten negative items i.e. Positive affect, Negative affect, Positive behaviour, Negative behaviour, Positive cognition, and negative cognition. In addition, five final items are added for construct validity.

Forgiveness is a 'process of letting go.' Forgiveness can be likened to a 'game' of tug-of-war. Provided that both parties on each end of the rope are tugging, you have a 'battle'. If someone lets go, the battle is over. If you decide to forgive, it would be letting go of your end; if you have released your end, the battle is over for you. In terms of letting go of resentments there could be an offensive situation that you have experienced; it does not necessarily have to be a person. Perhaps you were not sure who actually harmed you; this then moves into a situation rather than a person that needs the application of the forgiveness process. It is the letting go of negative feelings about the perpetrator or situation, and the emotional consequences of the hurt, especially the 'bitterness and resentment,' on which the course places most emphasis. You will be required to keep a journal of your feelings and to keep your 'EFI scores' close at hand. Keeping a journal is important. In smaller working groups you will be required to share some of the resentments that you have recorded in your journal. Items on the EFI will be discussed in a group format. It is important to note that if you don't feel happy sharing certain topics in the smaller groups, you don't have to. The course presenters will always be available for support and assistance.

Forgiveness

'If there are dreams about a beautiful South Africa, there are also roads that lead to their goal. Two of these roads could be named Goodness and Forgiveness. '
Nelson Mandela

To forgive means that you 'refuse' to retain harmful feelings towards a person or situation. In practical terms this translates into giving up the satisfaction of knowing that the one that caused your hurt will get hurt in the end. It's the quiet, silent, 'inner desire' for revenge that keeps anger alive in our minds and lives. According to the Oxford dictionary, the word forgiveness has several shades of meaning:

To 'absolve' from payment of (to cancel a debt).

To 'excuse' from a fault or an offence.

To 'renounce' anger or resentment against.

To 'give up' the wish to punish or to get even with.

To bestow a 'favour' unconditionally.

To release, set at liberty, 'unchain.'

Forgiveness involves a diminished focus on, or letting go of negative attitudes such as anger and hostility. Whilst uncovering anger, one may experience feelings of hate, hostility and bitterness alongside ruminative thoughts of revenge. Patterns of expressing anger vary with the associated negative feelings and a possible desire for revenge. The process of forgiveness starts with recognition that an injustice has taken place, and an acknowledgement of the psychological suffering. Unforgiving anger and vengeful fantasies can become habitual and very resistant to change. Depending on the level of the injustice, one is encouraged to reconstruct the anger evoking story, in an environment that is mutually supportive and empathic. During this stage of group work members are encouraged to develop new ways of thinking about the perpetrator. It is important to note that this exercise is not to help one develop new ways of thinking to excuse the offender of responsibility. Despite the recognized importance of forgiveness, the study of this important process has been relatively neglected by psychology. This may in part be a neglect of the positive aspects of life (McCullough et al., 2001). There seems to be a significant change over the last few years with a substantial amount of research published. From a psychological perspective, Enright's (1992) definition of forgiveness will be the primary framework used in this anger management and life skills course.

Over the last decade there has been increasing literature on interpersonal forgiveness from a range and variety of psychological perspectives. Bonar (1989) contends that the need for forgiveness can be explained within every major system of psychology. The overview of psychological understanding of forgiveness begins with the work of Enright and his colleagues at the University of Wisconsin where they conceptualize forgiveness from a cognitive developmental perspective. According to this model, forgiveness can also be conceptualised as an affect, behaviour, and a personality trait.

Enright's work appears to be the most comprehensively formulated and clearly articulated definition in the psychological literature. In addition, Enright's work has been published as a life tool by the American Psychological Association (Enright et al., 1992). The Enright Forgiveness Inventory (EFI) has provided a means of qualitatively measuring levels of interpersonal forgiveness in the affective, behavioural, personality traits and cognitive domains (Enright et al., 1992). Enright (2001) and the Human Development Study Group propose that forgiveness is the overcoming of negative affect and judgment toward the offender, not by denying ourselves the rights to such affect and judgment, but by endeavouring to view the offender with benevolence, compassion, and even love, while recognizing that he or she has abandoned their rights to them. Enright (1992) elaborates that forgiveness involves affective, cognitive and behavioural systems. This is how one person forgiving another feels, thinks and behaves toward him or her. (Subkoviak, Enright, Wu Gassin, Freedman, Olson, Sarinopoulos, 1992).

According to the Human Development Study Group, the most important part of this definition appears to be: the one who forgives has suffered deep hurt, thus showing resentment; the offended person has a moral right to resentment but overcomes it nonetheless. Following this process a new response to the other accrues, including compassion and love. This loving response occurs despite the realization that there is no obligation to love the offender (Subkoviak, Enright et al., 1992). According to Enright (1992) the psychological response that is forgiveness includes the absence of negative affect, judgment and behaviour toward the perpetrator and the presence of positive affect, judgment and behaviour (Subkoviak, Enright et al., 1992).

According to Enright (1992) the psychological response that is forgiveness includes the absence of negative affect, judgment and behaviour (Subkoviak, Enright et. al., 1992) Fitzgibbons (1986) reported that people who have a wide range of psychological symptoms could experience positive change through the forgiveness process. According to this psychological model the negative behaviour toward the perpetrator is replaced with positive behaviour (Studzinski, 1986).

Pingleton (1989) indicates that the choice in the forgiveness process is not to retaliate but to respond in a loving way, giving up the right to hurt back. The individual becomes able to deal with the hurt that was caused. It is important to note that people forgive and let go of recurring resentments at different rates, depending on the depth and level of the injustice. Some are able to forgive deep injustices in a few months; others may take much longer. People that have experienced deep anger and resentment have often reported that it is not caused by a single occurrence. People are able to forgive others at various levels and sometimes years later these uncomfortable feelings return. Surface anger can often hide deeper hurts, especially those retained from childhood traumas. This surface anger stops the person from confronting the source of the pain. Confronting the source of hurt or psychological trauma, could help to move to the next level in the forgiveness process.

Discover the Roots to Your Anger

Using Enright's (1992) guidepost for the process, the work draws on two important phases. Phase one includes engaging in the process of 'uncovering your anger.'

You will be required to answer the following questions.

How have you avoided dealing with your anger?

Have you ever faced your anger?

Are you afraid to expose your anger?

Has your anger affected your health?

Have you been obsessed about the injury of the offender?

Do you compare your situation with that of the offender?

Has the injury caused a permanent change in your life?

Has the injury caused a change in your world view?

The next phase in Enright's (1992) model includes working towards an understanding of your anger and dealing with resentment. During this phase you will hopefully discover that you are not alone in your feelings. This work will help you realize that although your anger is painful, it's not about pretending that nothing has happened to you. You will be encouraged to make a decision to examine any resentment that you may have towards others. In this process you will be encouraged to challenge your own forgiveness ability levels, any bitterness you may have and any deep-seated resentment that you are aware of.

Hargrave (1994) notes that forgiveness and reconciliation are sometimes equated. It is evident that both psychological processes are involved in welcoming a person who has acted unfairly. Laurite (1987) contend that forgiveness is a person's choice to abandon resentment and to adopt a friendlier attitude towards the offender. Because forgiveness is a free choice on the part of the one wronged, it can be unconditional regardless of what the offender has done. Reconciliation always involves two or more people: the offender and the offended. This course will focus primarily on helping you let go of lingering resentments that have caused you to feel angry.

It may help to think of forgiveness as a choice and a process (Bourgeois, 2001). We decide to make specific cognitive choices, which we then live out in the actual world. Even if we decide on this course to forgive someone for what they have or have not done, it may still take a long time to feel any different about the person or situation. This course will offer to take you to another step in the forgiveness process, as sometimes even while forgiving we can still experience many hurtful feelings such as anger and pain. Some people are only willing to forgive others if they are completely assured that the person they forgive will change himself or herself. It is important to be aware that the forgiveness process usually changes the person trying to forgive. The process can also help the forgiver extricate him or herself from a destructive relationship. As newfound knowledge becomes clearer, new perspectives about destructive relationships can be revealed.

Interpersonal impact

Ellis (2005) notes that each situation or person that you don't forgive becomes part of your daily load that you carry around. You can take this pain into every new situation and each relationship you have. As a result, you develop feelings of anger, bitterness and regret. You soon realize that wherever you go and whatever situation you find yourself in, the deep feelings of anger follow you around and become obvious to others, especially in the way you react. The way you react to certain situations will give you a clearer understanding about the impact lingering resentments and angry feelings actually have on your life. If you tend to overreact to seemingly simple issues then this may indicate to you that a change is needed. The important aspect in the process of change is that one has to arrive at the choice on one's own. A good example is when an insect bites or stings, the pain you feel and experience is intense and sometimes out of proportion to the size of the stinger. At first you simply recognize the hurt then shortly afterward you begin to realize the impact this sting has actually had. The sting or bite could represent the cruel unkind treatment or insult that has hurt and offended you. Now trying to dig out the stinger represents the psychological task of realizing how this one insult or cruel remark has actually pierced deep within your self-esteem and self-worth.

'The venom of the bite spreads into the surrounding tissues,' which represents the way forms of resentment about all kinds of 'emotional injuries' from the past continue to cause you major interpersonal problems. As a result one could take this resentment and anger into the work place, onto the roads, into our 'intimate relationships' or friendships, into college and into all areas of our lives.

Encouraging forgiveness is not denying the pain, but it may help you to make a much-improved decision to change. Forgiving is not pretending that we do not feel. Forgiving is not allowing yourself to be hit again or to be used or abused.

Communication skills and mind skills

'Imagination is more important than knowledge because imagination is what we do with knowledge.'
Albert Einstein.

Webster's dictionary defines imagination as "The power of combining former experiences in the creation of new images directed at a specific goal." A similar word for imagination is visualization. The world's top athletes use visualization and imagination to achieve goals. Top achievers tend to 'rehearse' the desired outcome in their own mind before the event takes place. There are a host of observable behaviours found in all our communication patterns and skills. According to research there appear to be five main ways of expressing a relationship skill. One can communicate messages verbally, vocally, with body language, by physical touch and through sending messages when not face-to-face. There are a further six main mind skills which include creating rules, perceptions, self-talk, visual images, explanations and expectations (Ellis, 2005). The course places emphasis in 'incorporating' these skills into smaller group exercises.

Calming Phase and Deep Breathing

Finding a place or time to calm down may be a challenge; however it is crucial that you start making the time to do this. Several influential writers recommend 'learning to relax' when faced with anger and stress (Moore, Adams, Elsworth, & Lewis, 1997). Promoting relaxation as a process to help anger is based on the understanding that behaviour is learned. People who have learned to be angry when upset can also 'unlearn' unhelpful ways of reacting. According to this theory it is not possible to be angry and relaxed at the same time. The relaxation process may dissipate the hurtful and angry feelings. Relaxation can certainly help you deal more effectively with anger.

Deep, slow and rhythmic breathing exercises will be introduced during the calming session. One of the easiest and quickest ways to relax your body is to 'breathe' correctly. Learning to breathe in a way that will calm you down is an art in itself. You will be encouraged to inhale slowly through your nose, until you feel your lungs are filled with air. When you are comfortably full of air, you will be asked to exhale slowly. This process will help you relax; most importantly is that you should exhale slowly and gently. As you inhale deeply, your chest and stomach expand, and when you exhale, they contract. It's important to develop a 'steady rhythm' with your breathing and you will be encouraged to breathe at the same pace, time after time. It should be noted that it is important to try and breathe in very deeply and exhale slowly at an integrated rate, to make sure that you are not inhaling faster than you are exhaling or exhaling faster than you are inhaling. You will be asked to count to four while you are inhaling and count to four while exhaling. Progressive relaxation in combination with music may be introduced from time to time.

During the last 15 minutes of each session, the group is asked to find a comfortable place to sit as images of nature are shown, accompanied by soothing music. With the aid of music, you will be required to bring into thoughts all the situations and people that have offended and hurt you. You will also be required to recall the word-technique that we utilized in previous sessions and to recall the positive word exercise that you completed at the same time, bringing your positive picture into your imagination and thoughts. This will require using your creative skills.

After a few sessions you may begin to feel its benefits such as feeling cool, calm and composed under strain. Some people feel sharper, more in control and more able to make use of their rich imagination and inherent creativity. Some people have reported that their problem-solving ability feels enhanced and more accessible (Moore, Adams, Ellsworth & Lewis, 1997). People have also reported feeling body functions improve, such as decreased heart rate and blood pressure. Others have reported feeling an 'increase in control' over their own lives. Some make use of this technique to overcome anger outbursts. During this calmness exercise, you may also settle down and experience quieter levels of the thinking process; recalling all the strategies that are taught on that day.

Music

Music has always been a powerful tool for expression and has the capacity to change the way we feel about ourselves and our environment. Music is an integral part of our life from the earliest stages of development. Pulse and rhythm are experienced in the heartbeat, breathing and movement. Certainly melody is created in our first vocal sounds through crying, screaming, laughing and singing. In our early dialogue with our parents we experience psychological contact and communication through vocal sounds covering a whole range of varied emotions.

Depending on the type of music chosen, music has a very calming and relaxing effect which in turn can produce positive physiological changes such as a decrease in heart rate and a slowing and regulation of breathing. Alternatively lively music that seems to tell a story may be beneficial due to its ability of grabbing attention and acting as a distraction. Both of these factors are important when treating anger.

Music has always been a major part of our lives; we listen to music in many contexts. We listen to music when we relax, when we are at a party or at the movies. It is a fundamental part of our lives. Imagine watching a movie with no sound track! It is difficult to consider. There is no human society on the earth that does not use 'music' in some way or form (Wallin et al., 2000). Every human society uses music to communicate; it has a great part to play in social and developmental psychology.

Music has an important process to play and, in doing so, can:

- Encourage non-verbal self-expression
- Promote the development of social skills (For example, listening, turn-taking, eye contact)
- Develop self-awareness and interaction with peers
- Help to establish relationships and provide a sense of belonging
- Develop the potential for creative and spontaneous play

Within the structures of music there are areas such as the perception of melody and rhythm and the formations and maintenance of musical memories. We can all recall some music in our lives that had a particular significance or relevance. During the calming exercise it is important to try and identify what music helps you to calm down and then to use this process yourself at home.

Music can convey feelings without the use of words. For a person whose difficulties are mainly emotional, background music can provide a safe setting where difficult or repressed feelings may be expressed and contained. Support and acceptance in the group in a constructive, musically-relaxed environment can help one to work towards emotional release and self-acceptance. Music is essentially a social activity involving communication, listening and sharing. These skills may be developed within the group. Over the course you may develop a greater awareness of your own anger triggers in relation to others. This can include developing greater confidence in your own ability to repair relationships and to find positive ways of making these needs known. It can greatly enhance your self-esteem if you are in a musically-relaxed environment. This also provides additional support when working in smaller groups.

Music is a great motivator and can be used to promote new ways of thinking. Involvement in creative music can assist physical awareness and develop attention, memory and concentration.

TECHNIQUES AND STRATEGIES

Consciously determine to be calm, don't react. Think first. Remember the goals you set in your anger management training and respond in an appropriate manner. Once you notice that you feel hurt, remember that you have a choice. You don't have to slide into revenge; you can choose another form of reaction that will be productive.

Ask yourself what your diet is like? Are you following the principles taught on the anger management course? Are you doing any exercise?

Assertive communication - one way of handling passive aggressive issues is to state in clear terms what you want from others and then ask them directly. Repeat this communication if necessary. Find out whether they agree with your requests and when they will be completed. This form of positive assertive communication has proven to be an effective strategy.

'Name the game.' With this strategy you are pointing out to the person what you are seeing and experiencing in their behaviour.

It's very important not to accuse them, but to simply describe what you are seeing and feeling. This encourages open communication. The blame game is an art of not taking responsibility for your actions

When feeling victimized or out of control, blaming can help us deal with past injustices, whether real or perceived. By blaming we are protecting ourselves and this is a maladaptive response. Blaming others prevents you from doing the necessary self-analysis, ultimately preventing you from moving on.

Taking ownership of your emotions and managing your responses to setbacks and minor irritations is the first step towards removing yourself from the 'blame game.' A good way of taking ownership of these emotions is to use 'I' statements. This lets the other person know about your feelings and makes it clear that you own the feeling of anger and are ultimately responsible for it.

Remind yourself of the positive constructive word-exercise you did on the anger management course. Each time you feel that anger arising in you start to recall the pictures you created with your imagination.

When the angry feeling strikes you, remind yourself of the list of feelings that you made in your anger management training and all the people and situations that have caused you pain. Work it out physically by screaming into a pillow, hitting a pillow, shouting at the top of your voice in a place where you don't disturb the public, or going for a good work out, run or brisk walk.

Acknowledge and clearly identify that you are hurt. In essence an angry outburst paradoxically hides your inner feelings of vulnerability, so you never recognize the hurt that triggers the hostile reaction. Not being able to accurately identify your hurt can lead to further bitterness and hostility.

The essence of taking responsibility is to learn to train your feelings to identify harmful feelings and then to manage them correctly. By abdicating responsibility we are telling ourselves that nothing is our fault.

In learning how *not* to respond in a defensive way, you need a clear understanding and description of the feelings that make up your actions. Remember that we often react in anger at someone for no reason at all; some trigger from the past may have caused us to react in a defensive way. This approach requires more problem-solving and less focus on who was in the wrong.

Holding onto anger can paradoxically give us a false sense of reality. It's a way of shifting responsibility onto others, and we end up with self-statements like: 'it's their fault I am like I am, because of the way I was treated,' 'I now have reasons to feel the way I do,' 'I deserve to feel this way.'

Communicate when someone upsets you. Tell them; calmly talk about the issue and the words that they used. Try and describe their actions. Better communication is the key. Don't jump to conclusions; when in a heated discussion, don't just say the first thing that enters your head. Slow down, think carefully, use the cognitive therapy technique and listen carefully to the other person before responding. Identify the thoughts that are causing angry responses.

Take a few moments to practice some simple breathing relaxation exercises, such as deep breathing, that can allow your sympathetic nervous system to calm down and dissipate.

Deep, slow breathing has an automatic physiological effect of helping you calm down, so when you deliberately take slow deep breaths, you are indirectly telling you body that all danger has now passed. As a consequence, your body will stop producing adrenaline and your arousal will cease.

Try to review your thoughts and calm down, as the first reaction to hurt is purely physiological. You receive a rush of adrenaline to prepare you to take action in real danger. When you have a short-term threat such as damaged pride, then all that adrenalin surges through your body and is not serving a meaningful purpose, causing you to stay in an angry state. Make sure you are not responding from your own hurt, but the situation as it is.

Remove yourself from the scene until you can respond without anger. Your final success will not happen overnight. Take it one day at a time. Your external surroundings or situations could be frustrating you. Identify the instances that continually anger you taking small steps to change the situation.

Take responsibility for your own life. You have to learn to identify your own hurts and stressful feelings on paper so that you can examine these feelings in a productive manner. The key to this strategy is taking responsibility for your own life. It will not help to say that you have put these feelings on paper and spoken about your hurts and agreed that you have forgiven everyone, until you have been honest with yourself and others that these feelings exist. Otherwise a shift in perception is not likely to happen.

When all the feelings of hurt have been carefully examined, the process of forgiveness can begin. Remember that thinking or talking through a secret desire to punish or hurt someone who has offended you can often be enough to help get this pain into perspective. This strategy is far more preferable than trying to bury these feelings deep inside, resulting in a low self-esteem and deep inner-guilt.

Remember the relaxation exercise we did on the course, and try to find music that calms you down.

Learn to forgive the other person quickly.

Follow and track the hurt back to its 'roots' and become more aware of its power. Failure to recognize old insults and past hurts can make the current hurt or insult seem much larger than it is. Become aware of how the past hurts can cause you to have depressed or angry feelings or low self-esteem. Unconscious resentment about past emotional injuries can cause major anger-related issues. Some people even suffer from mental images of revenge that are only subliminally perceived. Knowledge of the roots can lead to good mental health.

Use cognitive restructuring to change the way you think. When we're angry we tend to think in highly exaggerated and colourful terms. Try and replace these thoughts with more rational ones. Challenge your negative thoughts, as the way we think has a lot to do with the way we feel; changing your thoughts from a hateful negative orientation to a calm, positive orientation becomes essential in managing feelings of hurt or insult. Keep a thought diary and journal and revisit this from time to time, so that you can visibly see the progress that you have made managing your anger.

Be sure that it's actually anger that you're feeling at the time. Some people have such a limited knowledge of their emotional life that they tend to put other emotions in the same category as anger. If you examine your emotions more closely you may find disappointment, sadness, fear, or anxiety rather than actual anger. Don't confuse other underlying emotions with anger.

Use humour. Think up a silly scene or funny event to defuse anger. However, don't try and laugh off anger. Try to work on it.

Think about your reactions after the conflict or situation has occurred. Ask yourself, what worked? What did you do correctly? What could you have done differently? What could you do next time to make things go more smoothly?

Try and look at things from the other person's perspective. People make mistakes on the road; the person driving may be in a new era, may have been distracted or confused and is not maliciously trying to get in your way. Looking at the other side of the coin, or from a different angle, is called 'empathy.' This can go very far toward helping you to calm down, keep the peace and foster simple manners and genuine courtesy.

Accept your natural, healthy feelings of anger. Accept how you have handled anger in the past and learn how to handle the future. Remember the anger management course and make those changes.

Summary - Note from the Author

Anger is an emotion that is not something that will go away by itself. Anger when it is an immediate reaction to injustice is normal; however, it is in how we react that determines its influence in our lives. Anger is a powerful emotion that involves our feelings and thoughts. Unhealthy anger that is disproportionate to the initial cause is a major concern. Throughout our lives we may experience the pain of anger, in one way or another.

Using the word-identification technique, recommended breathing and relaxation exercises, cognitive behavioural therapy, diet, exercise, calmness exercises and the practical application of forgiveness in this anger management course, you may learn how to challenge your anger and to manage it in a competent way.

However, this does not preclude the fact that at certain times you will need to stand up for yourself, either to defend yourself or others. Sometimes you will be required to say something about an uncomfortable issue that most people don't wish to mention. This can be a reflection of your 'self-esteem,' and 'self-value.' To keep quiet and to try and hide your offended feelings is a slide back into revenge. Hiding feelings is not recommended as one tends to carry around these 'unhelpful' feelings wherever we go. Eventually we could end up taking out these 'hidden' feelings on others, for no reason at all. In my clinical experience there is no escaping the psychological effects of injury and anger, unless you take the brave step of facing up to the events and to start to forgive the person or situation. Revenge results in a destructive destiny. Each time that you feel injured it is important to speak up and share these feelings. You are then learning how to recognize your feelings and thoughts of hurt in the first place and make the changes. If you start to communicate with others, telling them exactly how you are feeling, this alone could set you on a path relatively free from angry outbursts. Some people however find being totally honest about feelings very offensive and will ultimately reject you for doing this. In my experience it's far better to let others know how you are feeling, than to try and mask uncomfortable feelings.

Tackling your anger in a group is a 'courageous' step to take, as we tend to act differently when we are with others. The presence of others while learning anger management principles can raise your motivation levels and help you address your troubled hurt or angry feelings in a safe, structured environment. Some of the goals in this life skills anger management book can help you 'discover' the roots of your anger. This anger management course may guide you through disputes without injuring yourself or others for that matter. The principles and strategies in this book can apply to all ages. The course attempts to bring you the understanding that you can choose alternative strategies other than revenge in order to 'defend' your identity or hurt feelings.

As stated this can be a long process. The human mind is capable of 'storing' hurt and resentments 'indefinitely.' On completion of this course you may still experience a lingering emotional arousal related to your anger. The key is that you have taken a step forward in the right direction and have made an attempt to take responsibility for your behaviour as only you can. The course carefully teaches you how to 'anticipate positive changes' in your life, so that you can experience life relatively free from anger. People have said that upon completion of the course they have experienced some important changes. These changes include: viewing oneself less negatively, viewing others more positively; some have reported changes in their reactions to unexpected events, people and circumstances in a much improved way; spontaneously feeling more 'grateful' and much more in control of stress.

I do hope that you will be able to affirm some of the changes that you have seen in others since attending this anger management course. To affirm means to look for the good in others telling them what you have found. To affirm also means to build up others and speak encouragement into their lives, to find reasons to praise others and to reinforce others to do well on their path through life. Find reasons to give to people to celebrate life. Working on your anger is one good reason to celebrate life, as you have taken the most important step. That is you have tried. One only fails when one fails to try! It is hoped that the cognitive behavioural approach encourages you to develop your own specific treatment goals, to think through anger provoking situations, and to monitor your own progress. Each successful attempt at managing your anger improves your self-esteem and self-worth. After this course you may be able to deal more appropriately with some of the inflammatory thoughts that plague our thinking by putting 'learned strategies' into practice.

References

Beck, J.S. (1995). Cognitive behavioural therapy: Basics and beyond. New York: Guildford.

Berkowitz, L. (1970). Experimental investigations of hostility catharsis. Journal and Consulting and Clinical Psychology, 35, 1-6.

Bonar, C.A. (1989). Personality Theories and Asking for Forgiveness: Journal of Psychology and Christianity, 8 (1), 45-49.

Bourgeois, M. (2001). Forgiveness is a choice. American Psychology Association. ISBN 1-55798-757-2.

Chen, S.C. (1937). Social modification of the Activity of Ants in Nest Building, Physiological Zoology, 10, 419-430.
Department of Health (2001). Treatment choice in psychological therapies and counselling. London: HMSO.

Dobson, K.S. (1989). A meta-analysis of the efficacy of cognitive therapy for depression. Journal of Consulting and Clinical Psychology, 56, 400-419.

Dyer, I. (2000). Cognitive behavioural group anger management for outpatients: A retrospective study. International Journal of Psychiatric Nursing Research, 5, 600-614.

Edmondson, C.B., & Conger, J.C. (1996). A review of treatment efficacy for individuals with anger problems: Conceptual assessment, and methodological issues. Clinical Psychology Review, 9, 250-270.

Ellis, A (2005). Rational Emotive Behaviour Therapy. In R.J. Corsini & D. Wedding (Eds.), Current psychotherapies (7th ed., pp 160-190). Belmont: CA: Thompson Brooks/Cole

Ellis, R. (1993). Anger: How to live with and without it. New York: Citadel Press Books.

Enright A (1979). Rational emotive therapy. In corsini, R. (Ed.) Current psychotherapies (pp 180-200). Itasca, Il: Peacock Publishers.

Ellis, A., and Harper, R.A. (1975). A new guide to rational living. CA: Wilshire Books.

Enright, R.D. (2001). Forgiveness is a choice. Washington: APA Books. Used by permission.

Enright, R., Gassin, E., & Wu, C. (1992). Forgiveness: a Developmental View. Journal of Moral Education, 21 (2), 99-114.

Enright R. & The Human Development Study Group (1991). The Moral Development of Forgiveness. In W. Kurtines, & J.Gewirtz (Ed), Handbook of Moral Behaviour and Development (pp 121-150) Hillsdale, NJ:Erbaum. Used by permission.

Enright, R., & Zell. R. (1989). Problems encountered when we forgive One Another. Journal of Psychology and Christianity, 8 (1), 52-60.

Enright, R.D., Santos, M.J., & Al-Mabuk, R (1989). The Adolescent as Forgiver. Special Issue: Young People and the Nuclear Threat. Journal of Adolescence 1989 March Vol. 12 (1) 92-98, 12 (1), 90-89.

Enright, R., Eastin, D., Golden, S., Sarinopoulus, I., & Freedman, S (1992). Interpersonal Forgiveness within the Helping Professions: An Attempt to Resolve Differences of Opinion. Counselling and Values, 36, 84-99.

Enright, R., North, J. Tutu, D. Eds. (1998). Exploring Forgiveness. Madison University of Winconsin Press.

Enright, R.D., Franklin, C.S., & Manheim, L.A. (1980). Children's distributive justice reasoning: A standardized and objective scale. Developmental Psychology, 16, 193-200.

Freedman, S.R. (1994). Forgiveness as an Educational Intervention Goal of Incest Survivors. Ph.D.dissertation, University of Winconsin-Madison.

Freedman, S.R. & R.D. Enright, "Forgiveness as a Therapeutic Goal OF Incest Survivors" (Papers presented at the annual convention of the American Psychological Association, New York, 1995).

Fitzgibbons, R.P. The Cognitive and Emotional Uses of Forgiveness in the Treatment of Anger. Psychotherapy 23 (1986), 600-640.

Gingell, J. Forgiveness and Power. Analysis 34 (1974) 179-180.

Goldenberg, I. & Goldenberg, H. (2005). Family therapy. In R.J. Corsini & D Wedding (Eds.), Current psychotherapies (7th ed., pp 380-396).

Grogan, G. (1991). Anger management: Clinical applications for occupational therapy. Occupational Therapy in Mental Health, 11, 140-169.

Hargrave, T.D. (1994). Families and Forgiveness: Healing wounds in the intergenerational family. New York: Bruner/Mazel.

Heimberg, R.G., & Juster, H.R. (1994). Treatment of social phobia in cognitive behavioural groups. Journal of Clinical Psychology, 55, 37-40.

Huang, S.T. Cross Cultural and Real Life Validations of the Theory of Forgiveness in Taiwan, the Republic of China. Madison, University of Wisconsin, 1990.
Kassinove, H. (ed). Anger disorders: Definition, Diagnosis, and Treatment (pp. 100-140). Washington, DC: Taylor and Francis.

Ketterman, G (1992). Verbal abuse: Healing the hidden wound. Ann Harbour, Michigan: Servant, (1992), 13.

Lauuritzen, P. (1987). Forgiveness: Moral prerogative or religious duty. Journal of Ethics, 15, 140-149.

Maude-Griffin, P.M. Hohenstein., J.M. Humfleet., G L. Reilly., Tusel., D.J. and Hall, S.M. (1998). Superior efficacy of cognitive behavioural therapy for urban crack cocaine abuser: Main and matching effects. Journal of Consulting and Clinical Psychology, 65, 800-830.

McCullough, M.E., Kilpatrick, S., Emmons, R.A. & Larson, D. (2001). Is Gratitude a moral affect? Psychological Bulletin, 125, 230-260.

Moore, E., Adams, R., Elsworth, J., & Lewis, J, (1997). An anger management group for people with learning disability. British Journal of Learning Disabilities, 25, 50-56.

Novaco, R.W. (1975). Anger Control: The Development and evaluation of an experimental treatment. Lexington, MA: Health.

Reilly, P.M., AND Grusznski, R. (1984). A Structured didactic model for men for controlling family violence. International Journal of Offender Therapy and Comparative Criminology, 28, 220-230.

Rosenak, C., & Harnden, G.M. (1992). Forgiveness in the psychotherapeutic process: clinical applications. Journal of Psychology and Christianity, 11 (2), 188-195.

Schmidt, T. (1993). Anger management and violence prevention, Minneapolis, MN: Johnson Institute.

Sears, R.R., Whiting, J.W.M., Nowlis, V., & Sears, P.S. 1953. Some child rearing antecedents of aggression and dependency in young children. Genetic Psychological Monographs, 47, 130-200.

Smokowski, P.R., and Wodarski, J.S. (1996). Cognitive behavioural group and family treatment of cocaine addiction. In: The Hatherleigh Guide to treating Substance abuse, New York: Hatherleigh Press.

Subkoviak, M., Enright, R., Wu, C-R., Gassin, E., Freedman. Olson, S., L, Sarinopoulus, l. (1992). Measuring interpersonal forgiveness. Paper presented at the annual meeting of the American Educational Research Association, San Francisco, CA (April, 1992).

Tang, M. (2001). Clinical outcome and client satisfaction of an anger management group. Canadian Journal of Occupational Therapy, 68, 220-228.

Tarvis, C (1984). Feeling angry? Letting of steam may not help. Nursing Life, 4 (5): 57-60.

Thomas, S.P. (1998) Assessing and intervening with anger disorders. Nursing clinics of North America, 34, 119-130.

Urban, H. (2004). Positive Words Powerful Results. Fireside, New York.

Van Balko, A.J.LM. Van Oppen, P.Vermeulen, A.W.A., Van Dyck, R., Nauta, M.C.E., & Vorst, H.C.M. (1994). A meta-analysis on the treatment of obsessive compulsive disorder: A comparison of antidepressants, behaviour, and cognitive therapy, Clinical Psychology Review, 14, 360-381.

Wallin, N.L Merker, B & Brown, S. (2000). The Origins of Music. Cambridge: MIT Press.

Walters, R.P. (1984). Forgiving: An Essential Element in Effective Living. Studies in Formative-Spirituality, 5 (3), 365-374.

Williams, C.J. (2001). Overcoming Depression: A five areas approach. London Hodder Arnold.

Williams, R., & Williams, V. (1993). Anger Kills: Seventeen strategies for controlling the hostility that can harm your health. New York: Harper Collins.

Yalom, I.D. (1995). The Theory and Practice of Group Psychotherapy, 4th Ed. New York: Basic Books, Inc.

NOTES

NOTES

NOTES

NOTES

NOTES

NOTES

NOTES

NOTES

NOTES

NOTES

NOTES

Printed in Great Britain
by Amazon